Homemade Sanitizer for Better Health

An Ultimate Formula to kill Germs, Viruses and Bacteria

By

David Nathan Fuller

© Copyright 2020 by (David Nathan Fuller) - All rights reserved.

This document is geared towards providing exact and reliable information in regards to the topic and issue covered. The publication is sold with the idea that the publisher is not required to render accounting, officially permitted, or otherwise, qualified services. If advice is necessary, legal or professional, a practiced individual in the profession should be ordered.

- From a Declaration of Principles which was accepted and approved equally by a Committee of the American Bar Association and a Committee of Publishers and Associations.

In no way is it legal to reproduce, duplicate, or transmit any part of this document in either electronic means or in printed format. Recording of this publication is strictly prohibited and any storage of this document is not allowed unless with written permission from the publisher. All rights reserved.

The information provided herein is stated to be truthful and consistent, in that any liability, in terms of inattention or otherwise, by any usage or abuse of any policies, processes, or directions contained within is the solitary and utter responsibility of the recipient reader. Under no circumstances will any legal responsibility or blame be held against the publisher for any reparation, damages, or monetary loss due to the information herein, either directly or indirectly.

Respective authors own all copyrights not held by the publisher.

The information herein is offered for informational purposes solely, and is universal as so. The presentation of the information is without contract or any type of guarantee assurance.

The trademarks that are used are without any consent, and the publication of the trademark is without permission or backing by the trademark owner. All trademarks and brands within this book are for clarifying purposes only and are the owned by the owners themselves, not affiliated with this document.

Table of Contents

Introduction

If you are interested in knowing more how Homemade Sanitizer will contribute to improved safety, and how you can save yourself from products that are unsafe and unhygienic, and making home-made sanitizers, this book has what you need. If you remain clean, it can eventually change your thought method behavior, how you will fix problems such as not having sanitizers in the market, and what foods and supplements are utilized that will have a beneficial effect on your skin and consequently on your existence. I have divided various sanitizers into separate types, and each sanitizer has specific ingredients i.e. Alcoholic and non-alcoholic, but it can have a major effect on the psyche, existence and attitude in overview.

Any men that are hygienic, make life seem easy and straight ahead. They easily get through the toughest days without breaking a sweat and appear to be feeling upbeat even in the most difficult of circumstances. These men are just the same as you. They express similar feelings and anxieties. Nevertheless, what separates the good and the poor is not genetic content or capacity, but their emotional wellbeing, brain development, and optimistic attitude to life.

If you have difficulty finding out what is sanitizer, how to buy it on the market, how to maintain yourself hygienic, how to motivate your wellbeing by utilizing sanitizers, how to steer away from toxic sanitizers, the effect of alcoholic and non-alcoholic sanitizers, the advantages of using a home-made sanitizer in your everyday lives, then these books can teach you how to resolve these hurdles This book will help you think about the sanitizers in greater detail.

Chapter 1: Effectiveness of Hand Sanitizer

Hand sanitizer, also known as hand antiseptic, hand wash, or hand wash, an agent added to the hands to kill natural pathogens (organisms that inflict illness). Usually, hand sanitizers come in the form of paste, gel, or jelly. Their usage is advised where soap and water are not sufficient for hand washing or where frequent hand washing interferes with the natural skin barrier (e.g., allowing the skin to produce scaling or fissures). While the efficacy of the hand sanitizer is subjective, it is used in a broad range of environments as a basic form of infection prevention, from day-care centers and colleges to hospitals and health care facilities, and from retailers to cruise ships.

The effectiveness of the hand sanitizer depends on several aspects, including whether the drug is administered (e.g., the amount used, length of use, frequency of use), and how the actual infectious agents found in the hands of the user are sensitive to the active ingredient in the drug. In general, hand sanitizers dependent on alcohol will efficiently eliminate concentrations of bacteria, fungi, and certain enveloped viruses (e.g., influenza A viruses) if rubbed vigorously over finger and hand surfaces for a time of 30 seconds, accompanied by full air-drying. Similar results have been documented for other non-alcoholic products, such as hand sanitizer SAB (surfactant, allantoin, and BAC). However, most hand sanitizers are relatively ineffective against bacterial spores, non-enveloped viruses (e.g., norovirus), and encystematic parasites (e.g., Giardia). Even when hands become visibly soiled before application of non-enveloped viruses (e.g., norovirus) and uncycled parasites (e.g., Giardia), they do not adequately cleanse or sanitize the surface. Even when hands become visibly soiled before use, they do not cleanse or sanitize the skin thoroughly.

Given the variation in efficacy, hand sanitizers may help reduce infectious disease transmission, particularly in settings where manual washing enforcement is low. For example, the introduction of either an alcohol-based or an alcohol-free hand sanitizer into classroom hand-hygiene systems was correlated with decreases in the absenteeism correlated with infectious disease among children in elementary schools. Similarly, the application of alcohol-based hand sanitizer has been linked with decreases in incidents of sickness and vacation days in the workforce. Enhanced exposure to alcohol-based hand sanitizer has been related to greater changes in hand hygiene in hospitals and health care clinics.

Agencies include the International Health Organization, the United States, Disease Control and Prevention Centers encourage the usage of hand sanitizers dependent on alcohol in drug-free goods. Indeed, the usage of alcohol-free products remained restricted, partially due to the emphasis on alcohol-based items from WHO and CDC, but also due to questions regarding the health of chemicals used in alcohol-free products. Work has demonstrated that the role of the endocrine system may be affected by such antimicrobial agents, such as triclosan. Another issue is environmental pollution induced by triclosan. Disinfectants and antimicrobials may also theoretically help establish antimicrobial tolerance. In 2014, the fears regarding triclosan prompted authorities in the European Union (EU) to ban the usage of the chemicals in different EU consumer goods.

By contrast, questions over the usage of alcohol-based hand sanitizer centered mostly on drug flammability and consumption, both spontaneous (e.g., by small children) and deliberate (by individuals pursuing substance abuse). The possibility of fire or contamination from unintentional or deliberate consumption of alcohol-based hand sanitizers is deemed small with adequate handling and policies restricting exposure to alcohol-containing sanitizer (e.g., distributing hand sanitizer to individuals).

1.1 Benefits of Having Hand Sanitizer at the Office

Many of the partners are coated with germs. It's not that bad; it's the plain truth of the matter. The average workplace is a cesspool with dangerous bacteria of all sorts, so that's why it's wise to hold the hand sanitizer still around! Will the sanitizer keep the workers healthy? If so, then how? Tell farewell to all sick days from here on!

If soap and warm water are not sufficient, there are also benefits of use hand sanitizer. You'll not only minimize the chance of illness, but you'll also transmit less germs to others and lose less school days.

If it comes to the ability to carry sanitizers around the workplace, figures don't lie!

• Sanitizers dependent on alcohol will raising the bacteria in your hands by around 97 percent.

• Proper hand grooming will minimize work-related absenteeism by up to 40%.

• Workers use a sanitizer at least five times a day at employment are around 67 percent less likely to get infected.

• Thirty seconds hand sanitizer destroys a ton of bacteria as two complete minutes' hand wash.

• Sanitation system offices record 24 percent fewer reports for preventable diseases by hand hygiene.

A few drops of a sanitizer for hands will function wonderfully. Fewer employees would phone in sick and a safer climate overall.

1.2 Hand Sanitizer Will Keep You Away from Getting Sick

Sanitizer may be incredibly useful for avoiding cold or flu if appropriately used. The more alcohol it produces, and the more often it is consumed, the less toxic microbes are on your skin.

There's plenty of data that this approach is successful. In 2015, The Journal of Occupational and Environmental Medicine published a report on the occupational impact of the sanitizer. In four years, six physicians collected data from various offices across the United States.

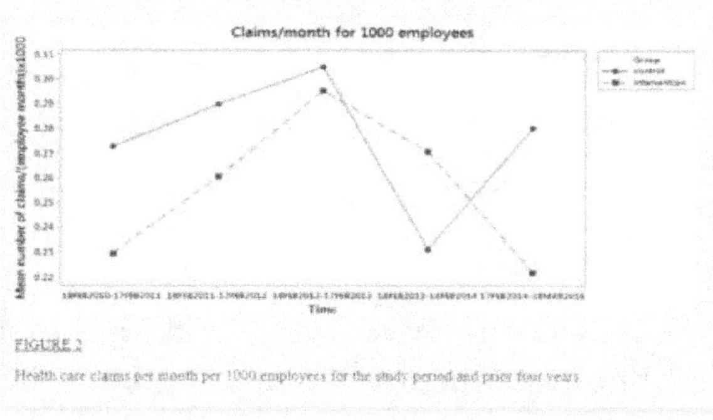

FIGURE 2

Health care claims per month per 1000 employees for the study period and prior four years

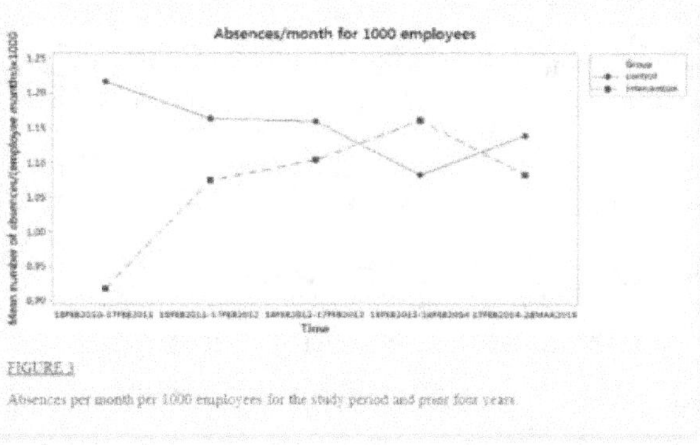

FIGURE 3

Absences per month per 1000 employees for the study period and prior four years

The Outcome? Health insurance expenses were lowered by more than 20 percent, and among the community who used hand sanitizer, the absenteeism was decreased by about 13.4 points. It is nothing short of an achievement. Employers spend more than $260 billion in health-related costs per year. Holding a hand sanitizer in the office sounds like a no-brainer to minimize the expense any further.

Plants may also help avoid germs from spreading across the workplace. NASA has authorized the following indoor air purification measures:

- Peace Lily
- English Ivy
- Bamboo Palm
- Chrysanthemum
- Potted Mums
- Green Spider Plant
- Gerbera Daisies

While germs may invade any inch of the office, there are a few safe-fire danger areas. Make sure to hold the hand sanitizer in the places below:

- On every desk
- By the doors
- In meeting rooms
- Near the elevator
- Outside the bathroom
- In the kitchen or breakroom

On Every Desk

You may think you have the world's cleanest hands, but germs crawl all over your desk. If you attach the bacteria to your computer mouse, screen, and phone, a total of 30,000 species would 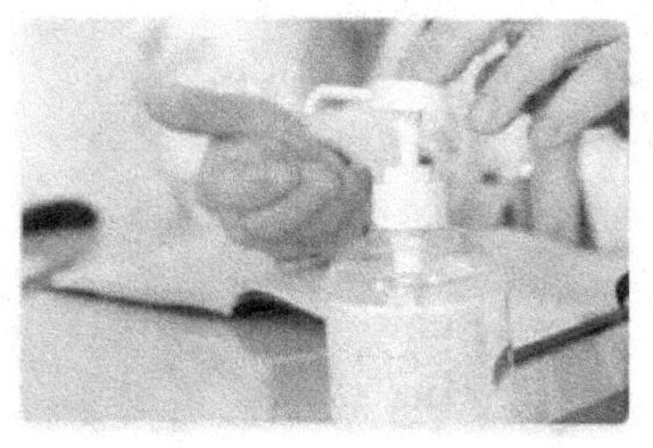 be present! Your strongest defense is a conventional sanitizer.

By the Doors

Doorknobs are no mystery to being hotbeds for bacteria. One germy handle could infect half the office within hours, according to CBS News! Your employees and 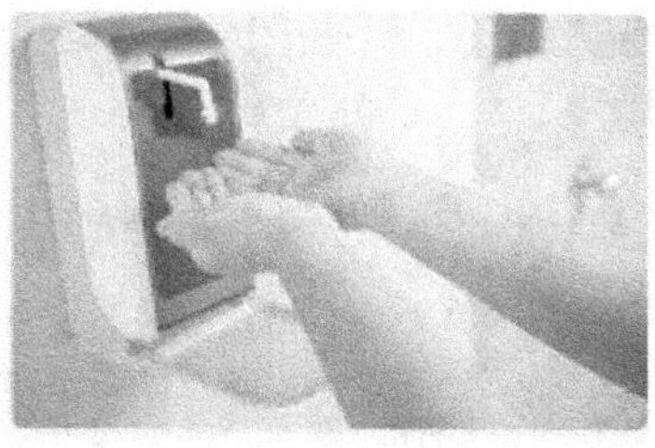 guests are more willing to use a sanitizer at the entry or exit, whether it is within reach of the head.

In Meeting Rooms

If Gary is in the midst of a highly stressful discussion, spittle could be streaming out of his ears. Cold and flu viruses will live for up to 18 hours on hard surfaces like the table in the boardroom! A couple of packets of sanitizer can help avoid illness on your squad. 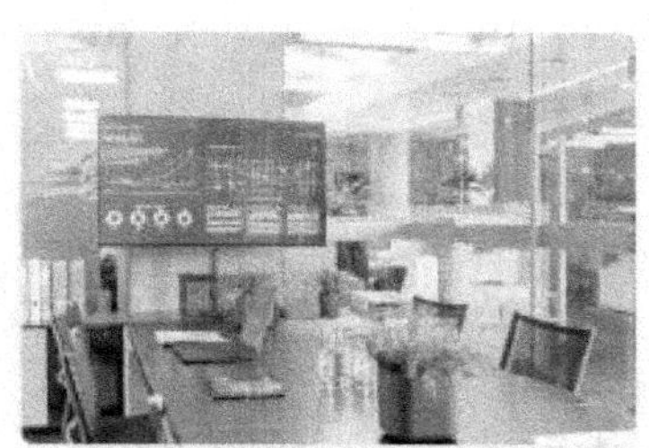

Near the Elevator

When they spit into their mouth, chew a packet of 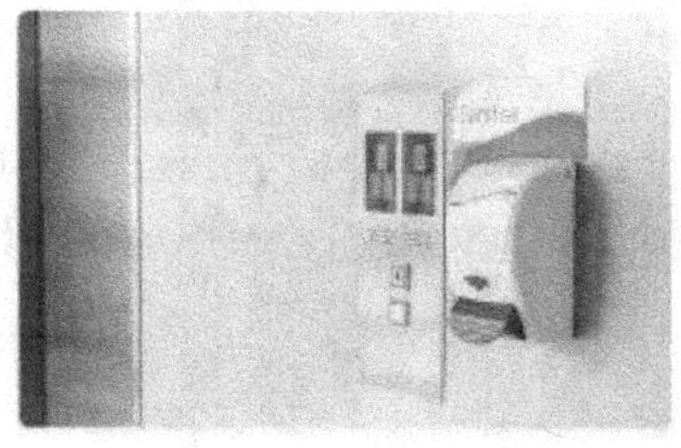

Cheetos, or use the toilet, the coworkers touch their floor numbers or the arrows. It's no secret that about 61 percent of elevator keys are bacteria contaminated. Do yourself a favor, and at each floor, put a sanitizer on a tray.

Outside the Bathroom

As cool as it will be to think that as you exit the toilet, the germs are gone, this is unfortunately not always the case. According to the research only 2-3% people wash their hands correctly. So, a sanitizer right outside the door is a reliable backup option, just in case.

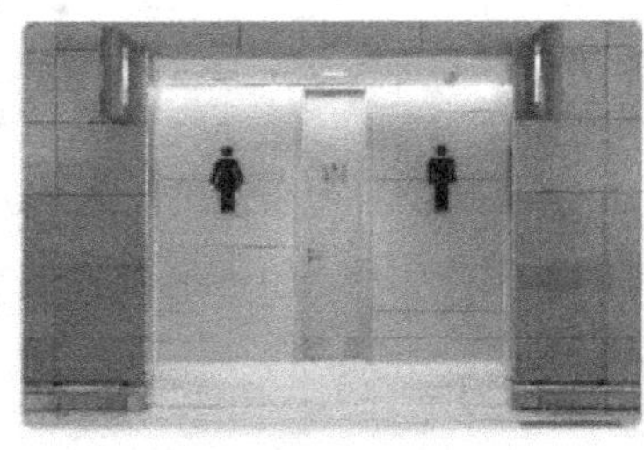

In the Kitchen or Breakroom

You may enjoy the wonderful sandwich because it potentially contaminates the office kitchen or breakroom. Most filled in bacteria are the sink faucet, microwave handle, coffee maker, and refrigerator lid. Make sure that you use the sanitizer before and after consuming your dinner.

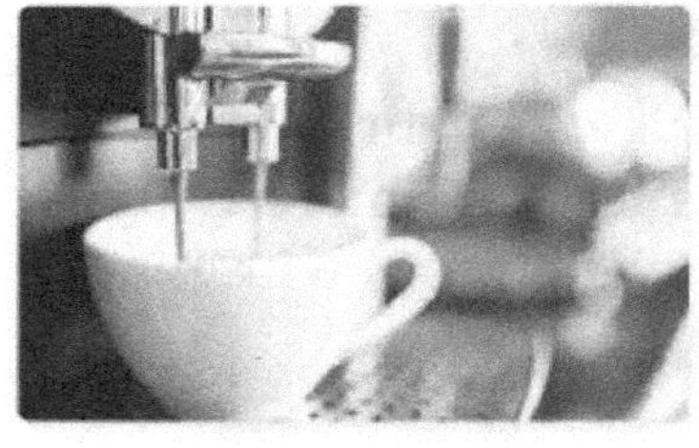

Hand sanitizer is great at fighting bacteria, but it can also be a fantastic way to publicize your brand. Customize a few little bottles with your name and contact details, and you have mini billboards just like that.

The sanitizer can be used to help grow the company at:

Trade Shows

A trade fair usually features big audiences, which ensures there would be a number of germs. If you sell strong sanitizer as prizes, your booth would be the one you will frequent.

Fundraisers

People at a 5 K, draw, or athletic event can pay for a couple of bottles of sanitizer. Using this as a means of collecting even more funds for the company or cause.

Grand Openings

Are you a new company in town? Give the audience a good picture of pocket sanitizers. When your visitors apply a few drops to their faces, they can wonder about your brand.

Community Events

If you're a small company, you may go for the announcement at festivals or fairs. Hand sanitizers are budget-friendly presents for stockpiling at your stand.

Ultimately, sanitizer is ideal for anything than just battling the common cold. It can also be a perfect way to put your company to more significant notice!

Beware of nasty germs and viruses; you don't want to get ill at the workplace. A couple of sanitizer bottles will work great, leaving you safe, balanced, and ready for a weekend!

Chapter 2: Types of Hand Sanitizers

The hand sanitizers may be categorized as one of two forms depending on the active component used: alcohol-based or alcohol-free. Usually, products dependent on alcohol produce between 60 and 95 percent alcohol, typically in the way of ethanol, isopropanol, or n-propanol. Alcohol rapidly denatures proteins at certain doses, essentially neutralizing all forms of micro-organisms. Generally, alcohol-free products are based on disinfectants, such as benzalkonium chloride (BAC), or antimicrobials, such as triclosan. The operation of the antimicrobials and disinfectants is both rapid and enduring. Many hand sanitizers often include emollients that soothe the flesh, thickening agents, and scent (e.g., glycerin).

2.1 You Might Be Purchasing a Hand Sanitizer that Won't Work

Germ X Sanitizer

Especially now, it's enticing to purchase one of the many hand sanitizers whose packaging promises it "kills 99.99 percent of germ-causing disease." But that doesn't guarantee the drug can shield you from the novel coronavirus.

The Centers for Prevention and Diseases Control advises brushing with at least 60 percent alcohol on-site sanitizers while you are unable to wash your face. Great pumps and bottle multipacks come off shelves throughout the shop. Yet "alcohol-free" goods— which the CDC would not endorse— still get snapped up in the marketing hysteria.

Some of the hand sanitizers are made by the Purell and Germ-X brands rely on benzalkonium chloride as the active ingredient, rather than alcohol. These non-alcoholic antiseptic drugs do not perform as well on certain germ forms, the CDC notes, or may merely suppress germ development rather than destroy them. Experts claim they might be more than none. Yet people purchase them without understanding what the difference is.

Such alcohol-free items are going out in full swing, despite internet price-gouging. Occasionally, from gazing at the lists, it may be impossible to tell whether they're distinct from the type the CDC suggests.

Purell Hand Sanitizing Wipes increased in quality on Amazon.com from $11.88 in January to $79.99 on Wednesday afternoon before jumping on Wednesday night to $199.99, according to the Keepa.com product tracker. They're all packed out.

The front of the box does not state whether it is alcohol-free; the back features a tiny print, whether it mentions benzalkonium chloride as the active ingredient and the "alcohol-free solution" name. This states it is alcohol-free nowhere on the Amazon product page.

Already sold out on Amazon is Germ-X Alcohol-Free Hand Sanitizer, with rates increasing from $10 in mid-January to $49.95 last Friday, according to Keepa.com.

On eBay, on Thursday night, six fluid ounces of Purell's alcohol-free sanitizer— the size of three-quarters of a cup— had a price tag of $55.

Amazon officials also confirmed they're tracking market gouging lists, preventing or withdrawing any they believe. eBay confirmed Friday that it is prohibiting listings for hand sanitizers, gloves, and disinfecting pads and that it would "quickly delete" listings other than books describing coronavirus or COVID-19, the disease it triggers.

If you type in Amazon's "coronavirus hand sanitizer," the results contain hand sanitizers manufactured by different firms that do not include alcohol in them. By the time of publishing, Amazon has not replied to inquiries about alcohol-free hand sanitizers.

Customers are puzzled. One offered Purell's hand wipes five stars with alcohol-free, benzalkonium-based chloride, writing: "Honestly, these wipes were a lifesaver. I purchased a kit because of the coronavirus and I flying to Vietnam... I used it on planes, utensils before feeding and seats before sitting. It brought me [a sense of security].

2.2 Alcohol-Free Hand Sanitizer is better

The benzalkonium chloride goods are better than none at a moment when all hand sanitizers are in low supply, says Emily Landon, an infectious disease expert at the University of Chicago Medicine. She said the CDC prescription for hand sanitizers is focused on the assumption that 60 percent of alcohol destroys "all the coronaviruses we care of." A benzalkonium chloride sanitizer as the active ingredient is "not as strong" since we don't learn that much about it, she said. She named alcohol-based items her "first preference" for hand sanitizers as a surgeon, mom, and infection-control specialist.

Labels for the alcohol-free hand sanitizing goods Purell and Germ-X containing benzalkonium chloride are unclear on the germs they are operating against.

ProPublica asked Kelly Ward-Smith, the spokesperson for Gojo Industries. This corporation developed Purell, what the drug labels imply when they claim they eliminate "99 percent of the most germ-causing illnesses." She declined to respond, stating in an email that because this article is regarding coronavirus, the FDA may view any reaction that contradicts its laws. The firm, which also offers alcohol-containing hand sanitizers, does not seem to be selling any of these for COVID-19 safety.

ProPublica contacted Vi-Jon, the corporation that produces Germ-X for feedback but did not get an answer. They often offer goods focused on alcohol; however, they do not tend to promote any of their hand sanitizers for use against the novel coronavirus.

Do not Waste your Vodka

The scarcity of hand sanitizers has driven customers to take radical action, making their vodka and aloe vera gel elixirs. Landon said she's noticed the "homemade Pinterest recipes" aren't lovely since people use whiskey or liquor that doesn't have enough alcohol to be successful. The standards for producing hand sanitizers from the World Health Organization include 96 percent ethyl alcohol.

Taking her marketing message to heart, Tito's Homemade Vodka warned her consumers on Thursday that her drug did not contain enough alcohol to efficiently sanitize: "Per CDC, hand sanitizer requires to provide at least 60% alcohol. The Handmade Vodka from Tito is 40 percent alcohol.

Chapter 3: DIY Hand Sanitizer Spray (Alcohol Based)

This DIY hand sanitizer requires only a few items and a few minutes to create. This simple formula for the spray sanitizer can be used on all hands and surfaces. Lately, I've noticed a number of Homemade hand sanitizer ideas crop online. Some of them are hand sanitizers manufactured with isopropyl alcohol, or even whiskey, dependent on caffeine.

I have been reading this quite a lot about the proper composition of sanitizers over the last few years. If you've seen any other DIY hand sanitizer recipe and handwashing tips as part of the free natural skincare mini-course, you'll realize that I've been using herbal and plant-based soaps and hand sanitizers for years to keep my hands healthy and keep germs away for our families. It's put handwashing into the mainstream withCovid-19 being in the headlines everywhere. The CDC states that the only way to prevent yourself from transmitting the virus instead of preventing communication with an infectious individual is to wash your hands and stop contacting your nose.

Thankfully, this has been my daily activity ever since my son started pre-school and began to come home with what seems like any illness known to man. Initially it was actually very hard for me not to catch any of them with a cozy and snotty boy, yet once I started to wash my hands regularly and didn't cover my face with my lips, it decreased the viruses I got by around 80%. This is also important to remember the social distancing, avoiding ill individuals, remaining at home if you're sick, stopping unnecessary travel, and utilizing alternate greetings (elbow bumps over handshakes) are perfect strategies to help prevent flu spreading.

3.1 How to Wash Hands Properly

I realize it can sound crazy to think about how to wash hands, but there's certainly a way to do things right and wrong.

I do use a good soap first. In our house, you cannot find antibacterial soaps, as I want to preserve the natural microbial ecosystem on our bodies.

Use Nail Brush

Nonetheless, I have a nail cleaner in my cleaning pocket. The toughest place to scrub on your hands is underneath the fingers. I do use such a gentle cloth. I use a nail brush to keep my soap within the soap bowl. This stops them from lying in a gloppy, slimy heap, which helps the soap to cure and last longer.

I purchased a set of 10 and gave them as presents, and I got four of them in my home, one in each toilet, one in the sink of the garden, and one in the kitchen. Atop each of those nail brushes is a strip of handmade herbal soap.

How to Dry Your Hands?

I dry them properly on a warm towel, after my hands have been lathered and rinsed. I hold a collection of wash-cloths next to the sink throughout the cold and flu season. They may be used to dry hands once, then placed into a laundry basket and cleaned before reusing.

Non-alcoholic hand sanitizer

I normally use my homemade aloe vera hand sanitizer mixed with thieves' oil while I'm out and about, a recipe that I posted back in 2015. Any time I shake it good, then add it to my hands liberally. So, I rub my palms together when I brush them, then attempt to dry them on a towel or a napkin. The hand sanitizer does not pretend to disinfect or destroy viruses but instead to mimic handwashing where there is no surrounding bath.

Hand Sanitizer Stockpiling

WithCovid-19 reports around the globe, stockpiling has also begun in places considered low risk. I am worried that hand sanitizers containing products that the FDA has defined as "not widely accepted as safe" are sold out entirely in supermarkets as they are hoarded by people and re-sold at exorbitant rates in second-hand markets such as Craigslist and Facebook.

I'm concerned about this behavior for a couple of reasons:

1. Such hand sanitizers contain ingredients that our bodies recognize as toxic. Their extensive usage is not inherently perfect for people. This being mentioned, I think there is interest in these technologies in healthcare applications where virus transmission is a far higher safety concern than removing the toxins from our processes. All members of the public should use hand sanitizers when entering hospitals and health care facilities, mainly where seniors and people who have health risks live.

2. Good people purchase hand sanitizer they don't require, but it's not accessible yet for those who are in great require.

3. Killing off 99.9 percent of all "germs" will not cause our body biomes to promote the safe micro-organisms that first help defend us. It relates to the problem of what we will open the path to by finishing anything off.

With all that said, I invented an oil-based hand sanitizer with oil for use as a spray on the hand and the floor. For the most part, I'm always going to use hand washing as my primary source to avoid the transmission of pathogens, so when I can't, I'm going to use this hand sanitizer product, focused on alcohol.

I assume we have sound immune systems at this time of year, centered on our balanced lives, behaviors, age, and herbal help. That said, not everybody is as fortunate as we are, so I intend to do my best to prevent other people so our healthcare system from being overloaded.

It doesn't suggest I'm going to depend on this sanitizer hand to defend myself and others. I should practice social distancing for more significant effect, avoiding sick men, sitting at home while I feel upset, and trading handshakes (and hugs) for elbow bumps. I also cancelled my book tour last week even though it was inside Canada and found it to be low risk. I guess the only thing that I can do now is to maintain some space to make the curve flatten.

3.2 DIY Hand Sanitizer from Alcohol

Let's focus on alcohol. The guidelines are that to be safe, the dosage of hand sanitizer must be 70 percent alcohol. I've seen different directions range from 60 to 70 percent, so let's only use 70 percent of our baseline to be secure.

That does NOT mean that the product in the recipe will comprise 70 percent. It says 70 percent of the language will be alcohol. In this case, vodka won't work since it's only 40 percent alcohol. I've seen specific formulas that include 70% isopropyl alcohol as only one component in a mixture, so, 70% isopropyl alcohol is 70% alcohol and 30% water (and other additives).

On its own, 70 percent of isopropyl alcohol satisfies the necessary specifications. However, this ensures that you cannot mix it with other ingredients to create an appropriate spray for the hand sanitizer. You use the 99 percent isopropyl alcohol to create your hand sanitizer. Instead, you should apply 29 percent of other ingredients, such as Aloe Vera, witch hazel, purified water, hydrosol, and essential oils.

Is Isopropyl Alcohol Safe?

The most widely used isopropyl alcohol is for sterilization. I use a tiny amount to disinfect my devices and containers while formulating lotions and other skincare items. These may also be used to cleanse wounds in healthcare conditions.

There are typically no health issues in limited quantities, but it may be harmful when inhaled or consumed through the eyes, and most certainly, when swallowed. Please do NOT drink it, and seek emergency help urgently if anyone gets it. Breathing in huge quantities of the gases will even render you sick.

It has a healthy level of 2 according to the Skin-Deep website, indicating it is normally a healthy ingredient, although it is noted that it may induce skin irritation. Using it on your hands would certainly induce dryness, and repeated usage may induce rashes and cracking of dermatitis. So, if you're going to use an Isopropyl alcohol hand sanitizer, please do it with care, and use it sparingly.

Where to Find Alcohol for Sanitizer

Unfortunately, there still appears to be a lack of isopropyl alcohol at the moment owing to stockpiling. You might not be able to locate it online at the moment, but ideally, it would be short-lived.

Attempt to search grocery stores, medical supplies shops, or even a pharmacy. Often, you might inquire about a convenience store or some other shop when their next drug shipment is in. Some shops will also hold a fair sum for you– to make many batches of this sanitizer; you'll only need one tube.

How to Make a Hand Sanitizer?

It is one of the simplest dishes to produce. I appreciate that this is also a spray sanitizer-it makes textures and hands even more simple to use.

A brief warning, before we get to the recycle. Both handmade recettes, including this one, were not checked by any third party and should always be treated with care as well. I propose spot-checking this mixture until wider usage to ensure that harmful reactions can occur. Though I always make every attempt to provide valuable details, any dependence you put on such details is at your own risk. This article is not a replacement for some form of medical, legal, or other qualified advice.

Hand Sanitizer Material

You need to make a spray of 100 ml for this. You should double the amount and split it into various spray cans, should you decide to produce more. I prefer to carry one at home and one in my bag. When you've got a baby pack, you might as easily hide one there.

- **75ml Isopropyl alcohol 99%**

- **10 ml Witch hazel or Lavender Hydrosol**

- **15 ml Aloe Vera gel**

- **4 drops each of sweet orange, lavender, and tea tree essential oil**

Weigh your Material

Weighing them is the best way to provide a reasonably precise calculation of the products. A basic kitchen scale, such as this one, is what you need. You may notice that it is much simpler than just using measurement cups. Using a funnel, attach all the ingredients with an atomizer cap to a 100ml container. Screw the cap back on, then quickly shake well to mix the ingredients. Making sure you give it another enthusiastic shake any time you use it, too. Whenever you are using DIY hand sanitizer spray (or any spray sanitizer for your skin), spray your skin so that they are fully coated, rub them together, and let them rinse.

Chapter 4: Alcoholic Sanitizer

Compliance with the guidelines on hand hygiene is crucial to minimizing colonization and inflammation of all people's hands, and especially the hands of health care workers (HCW). This would reduce the spread of microorganisms to patients, thereby decreasing morbidity, mortality, and the costs associated with HCAI. The global HCAI strain is massive. Statistics show that in industrialized and emerging countries globally, more than 1.4 million people are impacted at any moment. There is sufficient proof that hand antisepsis decreases the spread of infections, and the occurrence of HCAI correlated with healthcare.

Also, after too much focus on hand hygiene, recent reports indicate insufficient conformity with hand hygiene in the medical environment. In an emergency department's 2017 survey of healthcare workers, the approval rate was just 54 percent. The performance was also smaller in a sample of EMS suppliers on hand hygiene procedures.

According to the Center for Disease Control (CDC), hand grooming involves brushing the hands by using soap and water handwashing, antiseptic handwashing, antiseptic hand rubbings, such as alcohol-based hand sanitizers (ABHS), foams or gels, or antiseptic surgical palms. Alcohol hand sanitizers are being commonly used as disinfectants over hand washing of soap and water for many purposes. Their ease of access, no need for water or plumbing, and their proven efficiency in microbial load reduction are only a couple. In one research, a hospital-wide, hand hygiene program with particular focus on a bedside, alcohol-based hand disinfection culminated inconsistent progress in accordance with hand hygiene, coinciding with a decrease in nosocomial infections and transmission of MRSA. Promoting bedside, antiseptic, hand rubs has mostly led to enforcement benefits. Many other researches have shown that HCWs have improved compliance with hand hygiene by making bedside alcohol solutions accessible

Nevertheless, it is necessary to note that the potency of the alcohol hand sanitizer depends on whether and how much drug is used, the correct procedure, and the quality of usage. There are also cases where, for example, certain materials are not useful in avoiding the spread of other pathogens, or when the hands become heavily soiled, and the bacterial load becomes too large.

Non-Alcohol Based Hand Sanitizers

Benzalkonium chloride, quaternary ammonium, is the active component of most non-alcoholic hand sanitizer items commercially available. This is non-flammable and is relatively non-toxic owing to small amounts of benzalkonium. Such treatments, mostly water-based foams, are usually much smoother on the hands and tend to provide safety long after the product has dried. In cases of unintentional ingestion or as a possible fire danger, they pose far less of a challenge and are not hazardous to surfaces. Alcohol-free goods, though, are failed to achieve a foothold in the fitness industry. Most health agencies prefer alcohol-based gels, which are thus viewed as more reliable.

According to the World Health Organization (WHO), "an alcohol-containing formulation (liquid, gel or foam) intended to be applied to the hands to inactivate microorganisms and temporarily inhibit their development, can include one or more forms of alcohol, other active ingredients with excipients, and humectants."

4.1 Ingredients

Many hand antiseptics dependent on alcohol include isopropanol, ethanol, n-propanol, or a mixture of two of those drugs. The alcohol's antimicrobial function may be due to its capacity to denature and coagulate proteins. The cells of the microorganism are then lysed, thus destroying their cellular metabolism. Alcohol solutions with an alcohol content of 60 to 95 percent are the most successful. Notably, higher amounts are less active, and in the absence of water, proteins are not readily denatured. Alcohol concentrations are sometimes represented as percent by volume in antiseptic hand rubs but also as percent by weight.

Alcohols, including ethanol, are well-known antimicrobial agents and were first prescribed in 1888 for hand care. Ethanol (60 to 85 percent), isopropanol (60 to 80 per cent), and n-propanol (60 to 80 per cent) will reach the maximum antimicrobial efficacy. The operation is immediate and wide. Ethanol, the most popular component in the drug, tends to be the most powerful against viruses, although propanols have a more exceptional bactericidal ability than ethanol. None of the alcohols have demonstrated the capacity for developed tolerance to bacteria. The drug mixture may have synergistic results. The dosage of alcohol affects the efficacy with one analysis finding that a hand rubbing of 85% ethanol is dramatically stronger in minimizing bacterial species relative to 60% to 62% concentrations. ABHS also contains humectants, such as glycerin, that help to prevent skin dryness, and emollients or moisturizers, such as aloe vera, that help to absorb some of the alcohol-drained water.

4.2 Indications

ABHS is very good for the immediate removal of many contaminants by the action of the aqueous alcohol solution without the need for drying water or towels. Alcohols have outstanding in vitro germicidal efficacy against gram-positive and gram-negative vegetative bacteria, including multidrug-resistant pathogens (MRSA, VRE), Mycobacterium tuberculosis, HIV, influenza viruses, RSV, vaccinia, and hepatitis B and C viruses, according to the Centers for Disease Control and Prevention (CDC). The in vivo antimicrobial function of alcohol has also been reported in various tests, including efficacy in the elimination of clinical strains of Acinetobacter baumannii, methicillin-resistant Staphylococcus aureus, Escherichia coli, Enterococcus faecalis, Pseudomonas aeruginosa and Candida albicans from severely infected human volunteers.

ABHS is extremely successful in stopping winter flu, H1N1, URI, and other viral and bacterial diseases from spreading. Ethanol hand sanitizers are slightly more successful in eliminating visible rhinovirus, the most prevalent source of common cold, from hands than handwashing with soap and water. One problem is that the impact of ABHS on antimicrobials is quite short-lived. Adding organic acids to ethanol produced residual virucidal behavior that lasted for a minimum of 4 hours. It remains to be decided if such therapies can common infection with the rhinovirus in the natural environment.

The research reported in 2017 in the Journal of Infectious Diseases examined ABHS ' virucidal behavior against re-emerging viral pathogens, such as Ebola virus, Zika virus (ZIKV), extreme acute respiratory coronavirus syndrome (SARS-CoV), and Middle East respiratory coronavirus syndrome (MERS-CoV). It confirmed that both WHO could effectively inactivate all these viruses and other enveloped viruses. This also encourages the usage of ABHS in healthcare systems, particularly in situations of virus epidemic.

Another downside of utilizing ABHS is that the hands also get less annoyed. Too much hand washing with soap and water will affect the skin and raise the risk of infection. Drying hands with a towel first extract contaminant by contact during rubbing with the drying cloth and then pulling the moisture away into the tissue. Instead of unpleasant soaps and detergents, the CDC suggests using alcohol-based hand rubs that include different emollients and other skin conditioners as a method to minimize skin injury, dryness, and irritation. Damage to the skin can change the flora of the skin, resulting in more frequent staphylococci colonization and gram-negative bacilli. According to many reports, irritant touch dermatitis was lowest with well made, alcohol-based hand rubs containing emollients and other skin conditioners compared with other hand hygiene approaches. This extends especially to healthcare staff, which may wash their hands more than 30 times every shift. Nonetheless, it is understood that even items comprising emollients combined with alcohol will induce a momentary stinging feeling if the hands have some cuts or abrasions. Allergic touch dermatitis associated with hand rubbings dependent on alcohol is unlikely.

4.3 Contraindications

Some have addressed the issue of potential health consequences associated with accidental alcoholization (through inhalation and dermal contact) through repeated clinical usage of ABHR, indicating the need for further work in this region.

Relative Contraindications

ABHS has not been proven to be as successful against other pathogens as regular soap and handwashing with water. Alcohols, for example, have very low efficacy against protozoan oocysts, certain un-enveloped (non-lipophilic) viruses, and bacterial spores.

Cryptosporidium, a waterborne worm, is the main source of outbreaks of waterborne illness and is a common cause of diarrhea in day-cares. When contaminated, individuals with diminished tolerance are at the highest risk for serious illness. Hand sanitizers dependent on alcohol are not successful against Cryptosporidium, according to the CDC.

In the United States, norovirus is the main source of illness and outbreaks from infected produce. According to the CDC, norovirus triggers more than 90 percent of cases of diarrheal disease on cruise ships. Many norovirus infections arise as individuals who become sick transmit the virus to others. Healthcare services, including nursing homes and hospitals, are the most commonly recorded settings for norovirus outbreaks in the USA and other developed nations, especially in long-term care centers. Research has shown that ABHS is mostly inactive against non-enveloped viruses, including noroviruses. One study also noticed a correlation between the preferred use of ABHS for daily hand hygiene and an increased risk of norovirus outbreaks.

Nevertheless, also at lower concentrations, ethanol-based hand rubs have been successful against norovirus surrogates, when multiple forms of acids are applied to the hand rub. Furthermore, the potency of alcohol-based hand rubs against noroviruses differs from the sort and alcohol content in the formulation. WHO doctors often encourage the usage of alcohol-based hand rubbers during noroviral gastroenteritis outbreaks? There are differences too in vivo inactivity of alcohol-based hand rubbing against non-enveloped viruses. Studies also have shown that alcohol sanitizers decrease contagious titers of three non-enveloped viruses (rotavirus, adenovirus, and rhinovirus) and higher hepatitis A and enterovirus concentrations.

A new analysis showed that 80 percent of ethanol is impossible to completely kill poliovirus, polyomavirus, calicivirus (FCV), hepatitis A virus (HAV), and FMDV. However, the scope of ethanol virucidal behavior encompasses most clinically important viruses at 95 percent. Additional acids may significantly increase the virucidal efficacy of ethanol at lower concentrations against, for example, poliovirus, polyomavirus, FCV, and FMDV. At the same time, certain viruses like HAV might still be too immune. The problem is the tolerability of ABHS of higher concentrations of alcohol.

Alcohol gel destroys Clostridium difficile vegetative cell type but doesn't destroy C. Tough spores. In some trials, hand washing with soap and water was found to be more successful in eliminating C. Difficult spores from the hands of volunteers inoculated with a specified amount C than ABHS. Tough spores. However, there are no reports that have shown an improvement in C in intensive care environments. Difficult application of alcohol hand sanitizer poisoning or a loss in C. Difficult poisoning of water and soap. Wearing and removing gloves correctly in order to avoid manual infection during the collection process is of vital importance in avoiding C spread. Difficult infection and potentially negates any possible gain by using soap and water in hand care items dependent on alcohol. ABHS was found to be less efficient in extracting E as opposed to other hand hygiene methods. Beneath the fingernails, bacteria, and other microorganisms (caliciviruses). This is especially valid of longer nails and artificial fingernails, which reportedly contain more significant microbial communities than natural nails. Interestingly, a review of field workers shows that those that used hand sanitizer were shown to have increased amounts of urinary pesticide metabolites. However, this was not correlated with washing hands with water.

4.4 Technique

Efficacy is often strongly contingent upon the alcohol hand sanitizer application technique. The drug needs to be added to the palm and rubbed all over the surfaces of both hands until it is clear. Several experiments have been performed comparing the volume expected to be successful (2.4 to 3 mL is recommended), and the period taken for the application to achieve hand disinfection (25 to 30 seconds). If pressed just once, dispensers will produce considerably less than 3 mL of hand-rubbing, which would be inadequate to cover the palms fully.

In individual nations, foams containing 62 percent ethanol are used to decontaminate paws. They need a long drying period, which can limit healthcare workers ' enforcement while adding the required amount of foam. One study showed that the period required for the dryness sometimes surpassed the 30 seconds prescribed. Therefore, to improve the cycle, only a limited quantity of clinical practice is expected to be introduced. However, small volumes have struggled to fulfil the effectiveness standards and have become just marginally more successful than vapour.

Another study showed that high-quality hygienic hand disinfection is not feasible within 15 seconds and that ABHS is recommended for 30-second application time. Thirty seconds is a long period to wait before continuing with the operation one set out to do after disinfection, basically around the same duration as soap and water cleaning. The research also contrasted alcohol rubbing methods, including a 6-step process, and found that "good application" was satisfactory as long as citizens are made aware that they are liable for covering their whole hands during hygienic disinfection by hand.

4.5 Complications

Unintended paediatric ingestions are a problem about the usage of ABHS that is not an issue with soap and water. Hand sanitizers based on ethanol can induce alcohol poisoning if one person swallows more than a few mouthfuls. Around 2011 and 2015, almost 85,000 calls were obtained from US poison control centers about hand sanitizer exposures to babies. Some reports have shown that ingestion of ethanol by hand sanitizers in children can cause dehydration and hypoglycemia. Older children were used to drink hand sanitizers to get intentionally intoxicated

4.6 Clinical Significance

The usage of hand sanitizers dependent on alcohol has significantly improved conformity with hand hygiene in healthcare settings. They are reliable, inexpensive, and take very little time. While they might be less efficient than regular soap and water in some instances, if utilizing ABHS results in more reliable grooming of the hands, the trade-off might well be worth it. When it is recognized that microorganisms that are not sensitive to alcohol-based hand sanitizers or sides are deeply soiled are theoretically exposed, either soap and water (or both methods) could be the best route to go.

4.7 Enhancing Healthcare Team Outcomes

There's no doubt now that hand washing will be rising the transmission of several species. Hand washing is still difficult, though, and so the usage of alcohol sanitizers has become widespread. Alcohol sanitizers are used in health care centers and other sectors as they are more effective than only soap and water in destroying microorganisms. Many alcohol sanitizer formulations are available as a spray, paste, or liquid. While only do all health care staff use drug sanitizers routinely, they will also teach the public of their advantages. Alcohol will destroy much of the non-spore forming bacteria within a few seconds. Statistics suggest that alcohol sanitizers boost hand hygiene and can limit microorganism transmission in hospitals. Law enforcement is the main issue with the usage of alcohol sanitizers; thus, awareness and continuous reminders are required regarding its benefits. Nurses and pharmacists are in the unique role of educating / monitoring not just certain healthcare staff but also the public on the value of washing hands.

Chapter 5: Functions of Hand Sanitizer

If you haven't got the memo to wash your hands regularly, particularly now that COVID-19 is floating around, it's time for the soap to break out and clean. But if the Amazon prices give you heartburn, something that isn't as obvious is whether you should start collecting and stock up on hand sanitizer or even make yours. What are the experts saying, then? Wash your hands with regular intervals whenever possible, and if you can't reach a tub, the Sanitizer is also fine (both the kind you can get from the store and the kind you can). Here's the rundown of why soap first comes, and why Sanitizer's pros and cons. What are sanitizers, and how do they work? If you're so inclined, hand sanitizer is simply isopropyl alcohol, plus soap, plus fun-smelling essential oils. At first, the solution was used by hospitals and other healthcare facilities as a quick fix for doctors who did not actually have a second to go to the bathroom to clean between patients.

The way in which Sanitizer works is mainly through the influence of alcohol. By killing their outermost layer, alcohol will "murder" several types of bacteria and viruses, rendering them unable to take over a host. This isn't associated with hard outer shell viruses, including norovirus. Also, it will keep you safe in a pinch from a lot of the invisible gunk that you might be picking up on mass transportation or a public restroom. Soap works a little differently. Instead of destroying viruses and bacteria, their aim is to eliminate dirt, oil, and other hazardous agents that come into your hand.

Nothing is eliminated by Sanitizer: it only disinfects bacteria and viruses and can leave contaminants or spores in your skin.

Washing away the coronavirus may not sound as violent as stopping it dead in its tracks, but it has been shown to be more effective, particularly for mucus-wrapped pathogens. "There is nothing better than good hand washing where the alcohol really is," says Preeti Malani, a medical professor at the University of Michigan, focusing on infectious diseases.

I should wash my hands clean and use enough Sanitizer. Not really, says microbiologist, the chair of the department of microbiology, immunology, and tropical medicine at George Washington University — though continuously lathering your hands or dousing them with Purell, is likely to dry them out. So be prepared to be extra efficient when it comes to humidifying. "There is not much good in it besides that," says Maggirwar. To use the Sanitizer correctly, plop about three millimeters (about the size of a sequin) of the substance onto your palm and rub until your hands are dry for at least 10 to 15 seconds. You can do this anytime you like you need to. Just be mindful of alcohol's ability to dry. One thing that can be a bit tricky is that sanitizers or soaps containing ingredients such as triclosan can increase the risk of antibiotic resistance; these additives have not proven to do much to help your handwashing and sanitizing routine. Yet Maggirwar hasn't seen bacteria and viruses evolve to be alcohol-resistant or plain old soap. If you look at the label on your bottle and it says "antimicrobial," you don't have to turn it out, either. Using everything you can to stay safe and clean.

So, should I do a sanitizer for my own hand? That belongs to you. It's easy to make if you're using isopropyl alcohol and a gel-like aloe vera, and it won't be all that unique or different from what you can find in the supermarket. "Shake it up well, and that stuff should look and smell and sound just like Purell," says Jack Caravans, an urban public health professor at NYU. But be cautious about using more non-traditional recipes, such as this one which calls for vodka.

You want your hand sanitizer to be at least 60 percent alcohol, so you're going to need some 150 or higher concentrated liquor, says Caravans, not just your regular vodka. If you don't want to manufacture your own coronavirus killer, that's all right, too. "To me, it doesn't seem like a good use of vodka," says Malani.

Just be sure to keep your face and hands washed as often as possible, particularly after touching shared surfaces. Note also to periodically clean surfaces that are at risk of being sneezed on at home or office. Wipe down your cell phone, too, maybe wise if you happen to be using that a lot on the run. You can then shake your alcohol up for a cocktail instead of using it for your mouth and make it a little more fun to wait for this outbreak.

5.1 Difference between Disinfectants and Sanitizers

We brush up against a lot of misuse and misunderstanding between the term's cleaner, Sanitizer, and disinfectant in Nyco's neck of the facility's maintenance world. Goods can often be a mixture of two of the above, to confuse matters even more. For example, Sani-Spritz Spray is a one-step cleaner for disinfectants. N601 + is both a sanitizer for the foodservice and a disinfectant. And what is, exactly, the difference between these three product categories? In short, sanitizers eliminate bacteria on a surface by at least 99.9%, disinfectants destroy a wider and different range of microorganisms (than sanitizers), and cleaners simply remove dirt, dust, and surface impurities. Mentioned interpretation is very much clear.

But, there's a little more to it. EPA Certification Sanitizers, cleaners, and Disinfectants are regulated by the authorities like Environmental Protection Agency (EPA) and must, therefore, be accredited through a process that checks them to meet certain predefined requirements.

Unless and until it is EPA approved, a chemical substance cannot be classified as a sanitizer or as a disinfectant by statute.

(A chemical company such as Nyco may mark a formula as both, enabling the product to be called a disinfectant sanitizer.) Germ specificity All sanitizers and disinfectants have to be checked against specific germs. Chemical labels will separately list each of those germs. One disinfectant has the potential to kill germs X and Y, while another may kill germs Y and Z. It is important to take note and understand that not every microorganism will be killed by a single sanitizer or disinfectant and to know against which germs your products work.

Sanitizers are only approved for bacteria because disinfectants can also be approved to destroy viruses, mold, mildew, and fungi. Time to Kill One more aspect that is relevant when testing both sanitizers and disinfectants is the time it takes to destroy germs, and that always needs to be listed on a product label. Within 5 minutes, some chemical formulae consume respective germs and others in just two minutes or less. This is called "dwell or linger time" and should be taken into consideration when selecting and using sanitizers and disinfectants for different applications. Table Time 200, for example, eliminates 99.999 percent of bacteria * in 1 minute. A Note About Sanitizers is most commonly used but not always in foodservice environments. If a drug, like Table Time 200, is classified as a "food contact" sanitizer, it can be used safely to clean surfaces that will later touch the food. Food contact sanitizers should be applied as instructed and should be allowed to dry completely before the food comes into contact with them.

Cleaners Extract Dirt Cleaners, in comparison to sanitizers and disinfectants, are simple and clear! We constitute a wide category of products that physically extract dirt and soil from the surfaces using soap or detergents. Cleaning doesn't kill the germs; it just gets them out. There are cleaners from floors and carpets to vessels, for any surface under the sun. The EPA does not monitor or control the efficacy of cleaners. That said, cleaners certainly have different attributes and abilities, so buyers watch out!

Summary of mentioned things are, Sanitizers destroy, over a limited period of time, all bacteria and are controlled by the EPA, Disinfectants kill, for a limited period of time, all bacteria, viruses, mildews, or fungi and are often controlled by the EPA, Washers clear water, Make sure to use the right kind of cleaner for the soil that you need to scrub, Discuss your Nyco customer service representative or use the search feature at the top right corner of this page to scan our sanitizers and disinfectants for unique "kill reports" of microorganisms.

5.2 DIY Hand Sanitizer Recipes taken over the Internet

Unless you've recently cut yourself off from any news coverage on coronavirus (in which case, fair), you're well aware of the hand sanitizer crisis that is consuming the US right now. Drugstores and bigger chains like Walmart and Target have empty shelves where hand sanitizers were once kept, and even the prices of online retailers are inflated (mainly due to individual sellers).

The reality is that shortages are not entirely unjustified: while the Centers for Disease Control and Prevention believes that the very best way to protect yourself is to wash your hands frequently — for at least thirty seconds, and before eating, after using the toilet, and after sneezing or coughing — a second-suitable option is to use a hand sanitizer with at least 60% alcohol, especially when you're in the shower. But because at every given moment there is essentially a finite supply of hand sanitizer, it can (and will) run out — which is why many news outlets have started publishing DIY hand sanitizer recipes for this.

There are currently two key recipes circulating: one, which is "recommended" by the World Health Organization (WHO); the other, a recipe which the Vitamin Shoppe apparently suggests. Of course, it's a good idea: when hand sanitizer shops run out, you can just make your own — but is homemade hand sanitizer really as effective as store-bought, or could it be potentially harmful? Here's how to wash your hands, according to the CDC Unfortunately for the specific isopropyl alcohol and aloe vera industries — two products recommended for DIY hand sanitizer and sold out in many places — making your own hand sanitizer is not recommended for medical purposes. "For a number of reasons, we don't think it's a good idea to make your own," says Neha Vyas, MD, a Cleveland Clinic family medicine doctor, to Safety.

First and foremost, the proportions are all about a proper hand sanitizer recipe — and it is hard for the average customer to get those exactly right. \

Take, for example, the ' WHO-recommended recipe, ' which is less of a personal-use recipe and is simply intended for ' local production ' in ' countries and healthcare facilities. ' The list of ingredients includes precise measurements of three key ingredients — isopropyl alcohol, 99.8% (7.515 milliliters); hydrogen peroxide, 3% (417 milliliters); glycerol, 98% (145 milliliters); and that leaves much room for human error, to be absolutely honest. It would give you 10 liters of hand sanitizer, or just over 2.6 gallons, even if that recipe was made as stated and while some sources tweaked the quantities suggested by the WHO to produce smaller batches, that also allows a very real possibility of human error. The same goes for the other formula, of course, which uses a combination of aloe vera gel, essential oils, and isopropyl alcohol at 91 percent. In fact, according to Dr. Vyas, "the proportions in your little homemade laboratory may be off," rendering the product ineffective or harmful to your skin.

Another major red flag, the whole hand sanitizer argument is hygiene, which ensures that the devices with which you work must be sanitized, too. "If you don't use properly sanitized devices, you might contaminate the final product," says Ted Lain, MD, board-certified dermatologist and chief medical officer, and Sanova Dermatology. In addition to using proper and safe products, the WHO's approved "recipe" hand sanitizer also calls for air-conditioning and flameless production facilities (ethanol and isopropyl alcohol are extremely flammable).

Ultimately, according to an American Chemical Society member and former chemist, all commercially sold hand sanitizer products have been tested for their efficacy. "All you buy was through that [testing] process," he says, pointing out that home concoctions (and news outlet-recommended recipes) didn't, meaning their efficiency level is uncertain.

We know — this is all kinds of a downer, particularly if you went out and stored on isopropyl alcohol and aloe vera after hearing from the real stuff that your local store was out. But even if you have no hand sanitizer at your side, Dr. Vyas says that this isn't the end of the world. "Hand sanitizer is secondary to hand washing. The standard of care should be that," she says. And because (luckily) there is no lack of water and hand wash, you're always able to defend yourself against coronavirus to the best of your ability — even if you don't brew your own infinite supply of hand sanitizer at home.

As of the present time, the information in this article is correct. However, as the situation concerning COVID-19 continues to develop, after publication, it is likely that some data have changed. While Health is striving to keep our coverage as up to date as possible, we are also enabling readers to remain informed about news and advice for their own communities by using the CDC, WHO, and their local department of public health tools.

Chapter 6: Know more about Sanitizer

You squirt water, sense the feeling of the cold tingling, and scatter it all over your palms. Then, you sound soft. As an alternative to wash your hands with soap and water, it sounds pretty easy. It's quick, portable, and convenient, particularly if you don't have nearby running water. Hand sanitizer or hand antiseptic is an aid that arrives with products in gel, paste, or oil. Hand sanitizer also contains a type of alcohol as an active component, which acts as an antiseptic, such as ethyl alcohol. Other ingredients may include water, glycerin, and fragrance.

Many hand sanitizers dependent on non-alcohol include an antibiotic compound called triclosan or triclocarban. You may even use this component in soaps, and also toothpaste. Such goods are also called soaps, which are antibacterial, antimicrobial, or antiseptic. The American Food and Drug Administration reports that triclosan could bear needless hazards, including those on this page, as the effects are yet to be confirmed. Previous findings have posed concerns as experiments on the substance are underway on how triclosan may be harmful to human safety. If you're a cleanliness-obsessed germophobic who has made a routine of using hand sanitizer and lotion regularly, you'll want to know the hazards we've developed. Here are five secret hand sanitizer risks you do not learn, but you should...

Antibiotic Resistance

Antibiotics work against bacteria. Yet what happens if the body develops antibiotic tolerance, which in effect encourages bacterial resistance? Triclosan aims to make antibiotic-resistant bacteria. Using hand sanitizers will potentially reduce disease resistance by destroying good bacteria and helps protect against harmful bacteria.

Epidemic Intelligence Service's 2011 report at the U.S. Researchers from the Centers for Disease Control and Prevention reported that health care staff who were more prone to use hand sanitizers over soap and water for daily hand washing were almost six times more at risk for norovirus outbreaks, which triggers several cases of acute gastroenteritis. Overexposure to antibiotics or improper use of antibiotics may result in bacterial tolerance, rendering care more complicated or even impossible.

Alcohol Poisoning

Just because it has no triclosan, that doesn't mean it's healthy. In some hand sanitizers, an active ingredient is typically a form of alcohol that acts as an antimicrobial killing bacteria. The American Food and Drug Administration and the Centers for Disease Control prescribe ethyl alcohol, isopropyl alcohol, or a combination of all 60% to 95%. Six teens from California were diagnosed with alcohol poisoning from consuming hand sanitizer in March 2012, making it the latest in a line of household items known to cause intoxication, ABC News confirmed. A couple of hand sanitizer squirts may be equivalent to a couple of shots of hard liquor. Yet they are not all adolescents. This was in the past, mistakenly swallowed by smaller students, according to the LA Times.

Hormone Disruption

Another consequence of triclosan is issues with the hormones. The FDA says evidence indicates that triclosan can contribute to hormonal disturbance and allow bacteria to respond to its antimicrobial properties, producing more strains that are immune to antibiotics. Animal experiments have demonstrated that the compound could alter the way hormones function in the body, pose questions, and require more study to understand further how they could impact humans.

Weaker Immune System

Studies also have shown that triclosan can weaken the immune system as well, which defends the body from disease. Researchers at the UMS of Public Health noticed that triclosan could adversely affect immune function in humans. Compromising the immune system will render people more prone to asthma, and more vulnerable to the plastics-based toxic chemical Bisphenol A. Kids and teenagers with elevated triclosan levels were more inclined to be infected with hay fever and other allergies in the study. When your hand sanitizer is fragrant, it's typically filled with poisonous chemicals. Companies are not forced to reveal the products that make up their hidden scents and are thus produced from thousands of chemicals in total. Synthetic fragrances include phthalates, which are endocrine disrupters that resemble hormones and that influence the production of genitalia. You will also check for parabens that are found in several skincare items. These are used to conserve certain products, and to prolong the shelf life of a drug.

6.1 Things You Didn't Know About Sanitizer

There are a variety of fascinating details about hand sanitizers, theories and assumptions. Since many people doubt about the real usefulness of these items, some of these interesting findings are certainly worth thinking about. Everybody needs to remain clean after all, to make sure they protect off germs to diseases.

1. Hand Sanitizer Don't Create Bacteria

A fascinating misconception that many still claims is that hand sanitizers will potentially create excellent drug-resistant bacteria. That is obviously not valid as long as alcohol is the product's primary component. Of starters, the Honest Company maintains that it utilizes at least the usual 60 per cent alcohol products and offers hand sanitizers that are outstanding of ensuring personal hygiene; in fact, they conform to the highest requirements established by health agencies and organizations. There is no indication that the bacteria are capable of establishing alcohol tolerance. In reality it has been proven that alcohol-based hand sanitizers destroy drug-resistant bacteria. Of course, you do need to be vigilant of hand sanitizers focused on water and non-alcohol and make sure to review the bottle carefully.

2. Dosage and Ingredients Both Matter

Speaking of the products used in hand sanitizers, perhaps the only thing that counts is what is in your favorite formula. Of course, as stated, you want at least 60 per cent alcohol to get a sanitizer. According to Parents Magazine, anything less than this won't be successful and can potentially allow bacteria to develop. Yet you do ought to be cautious on how many you're using. The correct dosage is around a dollop of a quarter to a half-dollar scale. This would serve to cover the whole hands full. Having a little bit under the nails is always good.

3. Hand Sanitizers are Safe for Babies

Babies have very fragile and sensitive hands, but it doesn't mean they won't be able to profit from the hand sanitizers. Although the risk of alcohol consumption is relatively high, babies and even small children under the age of 6 barely show any significant consequences from exposure. Also, you don't want to overdo it of course. Make sure you are utilizing minimal doses of hand sanitizer, and your kids will be safe.

4. Hand Sanitizers Help to Protect Against Flu

According to the Product Search page, hand sanitizers will of course destroy a substantial portion of the flu virus on the hands and also reduce the spread of gastrointestinal diseases. However, there are also limitations on this. Hand sanitizers provide decent, but not absolute, safety since the flu virus is airborne. While using a hand sanitizer to remove germs and viruses will be a part of your everyday health-conscious practice, make sure it's not the only thing you're doing. Germs are everywhere; security needs to be multi-faceted and cover on the body not just the hands but also the neck and other places too.

5. Soap and water Doesn't Eliminate More Germs

Must you sanitize or wash your hands? That is a query that you may pose. When the hands are obviously sticky, so the better solution is simply the soap and wash. Hand sanitizers don't say much for real water. The strength of hand sanitizers is the idea they are designed to remove hidden germs. In reality, there have been more than 20 studies conducted by the Centers for Disease Control which show that hand sanitizers based on alcohol actually remove more germs than soap and water.

6. Hand Sanitizers Don't Irritate Skin

The reality is that skin reaction to hand sanitizers are very uncommon, even though they do have alcohol in them. Using a variety of specific ingredients such as emollients successfully soothes and protects the scalp. Experts also tend to believe that sanitizers are much softer on the hands than water and soap. Using a hand sanitizer appears to bring more moisture back onto the Skin compared to just soap and water. This is not a replacement for some other skincare that is already being used, but it is good to learn; they will also benefit.

7. Difference Between Homemade and Store Brands

Most citizens consider themselves under the impression that they may quickly create their own hand sanitizer. This is not valid, at least not a formulation or blend that should be considered successful. Perhaps a hand sanitizer ought to have an alcohol level of at least 60 percent. To be able to do this with a home-made product is quite challenging. If you want the greatest performance, keep away from home-made stuff.

8. Use of Hand Sanitizer as Deodorant

The hand sanitizer may be used as a substitute just in case you do lose your deodorant. The alcohol in the sanitizer destroys the odor-causing bacteria under the neck. Plus, the alcohol quickly dries up, and there's no risk of lingering wetness. The scent of alcohol often dissipates relatively quickly. Only don't do every day, as it could dry out the Skin of the underarm and cause discomfort.

Staying up-to-date and educated of these fun and fascinating details or misunderstandings surrounding hand sanitizers will help you remain healthier. Only keep your hands clean frequently and obey specific normal protocols to keep yourself and others free from harmful germs.

6.2 The Importance of Hand Sanitizer at Workplace

Employees use their hands during every given workday to compose a paper, shake hands with a potential customer, unlock doors, and many more. Both behaviors expose hands to toxic microbes and germs. Illness is related to a lack of efficiency, losing an estimated U.S. $225.8 billion to employers. Given that 80 percent of all diseases are hand borne, a successful hand hygiene system at work is important to enforce. Americans expend more time at the office Monday through Friday than anywhere, even at home. For a fact, except though they are injured, 90 percent of the office staff would come to work, partially due to an ever-growing workload. It renders the place of employment a hotbed for microbes and germs. A year, according to the CDC, flu costs employers $10.4 billion in direct expenses for adult hospitalizations and clinic services. And this year's gripping season could be worse than average as experts warn that this year's gripping vaccination can only be successful by 10 percent.

The Bonne News? Compliance with proper hand grooming will minimize by 40 percent absenteeism and related costs. Although, washing hands with water and soap is the safest way to ensure proper cleaning of hands and getting rid of germs, it is not always a feasible choice. There's one easy remedy, though: hand sanitizer. Hand sanitizer is one of the strongest methods used to stop being infected and transmitting germs, according to the World Health Organization (WHO) and the CDC. You will empower workers to enhance their hand hygiene and render the workplace a safer workplace by putting hand sanitizer in specific positions in the workplace and other high-traffic places.

6.3 Key Locations for Hand Sanitizer

Organizations encouraging the daily usage of hand sanitizer appear to provide more active staff. Research in BMC Infectious Diseases showed that office employees who were advised to use an alcohol-based hand sanitizer at least five times a day were almost two-thirds less likely to get sick than those who stopped washing their hands.

A study conducted in 2016 showed that while 92 percent of Americans think it is necessary to wash hands after using a public toilet, just 66 percent of them do. About one-third of survey respondents acknowledged that they should miss soap and rinse with water. This makes the availability of a hand sanitizer in the bathroom extra essential. When workers are in a hurry and don't care about halting and rinsing with soap and water, having a contingency solution at sinks and doors means the germs don't enter the toilet.

The easiest way to inform staff about using a hand sanitizer is to make it easy to use and always in reach. Placing hand sanitizer near and around high-touch surfaces and public areas is important, including:

Entrances and exits

A single doorknob could theoretically be the source of widespread workplace illness. In reality, recent research has shown that 40 to 60 percent of staff and visitors inside the facility picked up a virus put on a doorknob inside two to four hours. As well as routinely disinfecting doorknobs, light switches and other high-touch surfaces inside the office, ensuring that a nearby hand sanitizing station is often given to minimize the spread of contamination.

Cafeterias and Common Rooms

So, if food is consumed with germ-ridden lips, it's simple to ingest the germs and get sick with a variety of diseases. The breakroom and kitchen were one of the germiest hotspots in an area, according to a report by NSF International. Although hand sanitizer is no replacement for someone cooking food, it will help remove those germs.

Meeting Rooms

Meeting rooms are frequently filled with staff, clients, and other guests who share handshakes and transfer germs as a result. Through having an easy-to-access hand sanitizing station for visitors and staff, either at the door or the seat, it helps them to shield their hands from germs before and after the conference.

Employee Desk

Since we contact them too much, tables, computers, electronic keys, and machine mice are essential sources of transmission of germs. Considering that workers spend much of their day at their offices, where they also feed, drink, and sometimes cough and sneeze, offices are a "virus minefield" that can live up to three days on a surface. Placing individual hand sanitizers at desks can hold the safety of hands within control.

High Traffic Areas

It's also necessary to have hand sanitizer outside of the workplace. High-traffic areas such as airline airports, shopping rooms, and leisure facilities can provide stations for hand hygiene to ensure tourists remain as safe as they can. It not only leaves high-traffic places safe but also serves to boost the appearance of the city, store, or rec-center.

Transaction Counters

The researchers swabbed $1 bills from a bank in a 2017 report and discovered hundreds of species of micro-organisms live on them. Further work has established pathogenic agents such as E. Coli, salmonella, and staphylococcus aureus on paper currency, both of which can cause severe illness. Cleaning your hands after handling currency, particularly if you're about to eat food soon afterward, is crucial. Holding hand sanitizer around checkout locations, such as the checkout counter at the cafeteria, allows people to indulge in hand hygiene where it is most important.

Selecting the Right-Hand Sanitizer

Although supplying hand sanitizer at crucial office locations is important in reducing employee sickness and absenteeism, the safest approach to have the correct form of sanitizer is to do so. Be sure you use a hand sanitizer dependent on alcohol that includes at least 70 percent alcohol. The higher concentration of alcohol would normally turn into better effectiveness. Look for goods with a minimum kill rate of 5 logs (99.999 percent)–100 times more effective than sanitizers with 3 logs (99.9 percent).

Consider utilizing foam hand sanitizers, as 84 percent of adults prefer foam sanitizer to sticky soap. It is often safer to use sanitizers that include moisturizers to avoid skin dryness and to minimize possible allergic reactions and skin irritations; they are solvent-free and dye-free.

Encouraging the Hand-Hygiene

A full system of hand grooming goes farther than having the correct items. Although it is important to enhance the wellbeing of the employees to provide wall-mounted hand sanitizing dispensers and bottles on surfaces in and around germ hotspots, it is only helpful if the staff routinely using such.

Provide posters, flyers, internal newsletters, and information boards with reminders to clean hands near dispensers, and provide simple, easy hand hygiene details. These instructions will also give guidance on how to correctly use and administer hand sanitizer according to the World Health Organization's suggested 6 Phase Process, to ensure that the right quantity is used and applied to cover both surfaces with both hands. Furthermore, companies can give year-round training workshops and gatherings to educate and inform workers of how better practices of hand hygiene will enhance their health.

It is necessary, as an employer, to lead change with an example. Encourage employees to always use a sanitizer by doing it themselves. In the cold and flu season, do not neglect to load up with hand care refills. Eventually, advising employees to take a sick day when appropriate to keep the germs away from the workplace and all healthier staff is crucial.

Sanitizing the Workplace

Using hand sanitizer decreases microbial numbers and destroys other infectious germs that may affect flu staff and other viruses. This is important that workers take into consideration the wellbeing of their staff to make the workforce a safe and productive atmosphere. Having workers with a hand sanitizer, at desks, and in public rooms, is almost as important as having the appropriate equipment and resources for their jobs.

Conclusion

Hand hygiene is one of the major facets of increasing fecal-oral transmission of infectious agents. Therefore, differing hand hygiene standards for specific settings cause confusion within the general public as to what is the correct approach to follow or what products should be used for daily hand washing and hand hygiene. This guide provides the information required for everyday consumers to take informed decisions. Most people neglect that they ought to clean their immediate environment from the germs. This can only be done in a true germ-free environment in a laboratory or other medical space, though. We live in a dynamic world full of microorganisms, breathing beings that are unnoticed by our naked eyes. While some of the micro-organisms that cause illness or sickness, some can be essential to our safety and environment. While certain microbes that cause food spoilage or disease, others are a natural part of our environments and foods. Your normal meat, sauerkraut or other medications deficient in good bacteria would be missing! Without healthy microbial allies, cows cannot use the grasses for feeding. Therefore, without safe bacteria or fungus, our planet would be full of yard waste and other agricultural trash. In reality, we shouldn't neglect the idea that our normal, healthy body has specific external defenses and internal systems (immune system) to combat germs, as long as their numbers don't daunt. Knowing and learning how to treat or cope with both the good and negative microorganisms on our bodies and in our environment would therefore allow us to make efficient use of such microbes, thus the spread of communicable diseases. The goal is to reduce the number of bad microbes to a low enough level for the body to use the new immune response to fight them off equally.

References

- Miles, A. A., Misra, S. S., & Irwin, J. O. (1938). The estimation of the bactericidal power of the blood. *Epidemiology & Infection*, 38(6), 732-749.

- Yildirim, A., OKTAY, M., & BİLALOĞLU, V. (2001). The antioxidant activity of the leaves of Cydonia vulgaris. *Turkish Journal of Medical Sciences*, 31(1), 23-27.

- Rubilar, M., Pinelo, M., Shene, C., Sineiro, J., & Nuñez, M. J. (2007). Separation and HPLC-MS identification of phenolic antioxidants from agricultural residues: almond hulls and grape pomace. *Journal of agricultural and food chemistry*, 55(25), 10101-10109.

- Sharma, A., Yadav, R., Gudha, V., Soni, U. N., & Patel, J. R. (2016). Formulation and evaluation of herbal hand wash. *World Journal of Pharmcay and Pharmaceutical Sciences*, 5(3), 675-683.

- Ghasemi, E., Golshahi, H., Ghasemi, E., & Mehranzade, E. (2011). Antibacterial activity of Ocimum sanctum extract against E. coli, S. aureus and P. aeruginosa. *Clinical Biochemistry*, 13(44), S352.

- Dutra, R. C., Leite, M. N., & Barbosa, N. R. (2008). Quantification of phenolic constituents and antioxidant activity of Pterodon emarginatus vogel seeds. *International Journal of Molecular Sciences*, 9(4), 606-614.

- Larson, E., Mayur, K., & Laughon, B. A. (1989). Influence of two handwashing frequencies on reduction in colonizing flora with three handwashing products used by health care personnel. *American journal of infection control*, 17(2), 83-88.

- Kolhapure, S. A. (2004). Evaluation of the antimicrobial efficacy and safety of purehands herbal hand sanitizer in hand hygiene and on inanimate objects. *Antiseptic, 101*(2), 55-57.

- Kolhapure, S. A. (2004). Evaluation of the antimicrobial efficacy and safety of purehands herbal hand sanitizer in hand hygiene and on inanimate objects. *Antiseptic, 101*(2), 55-57.

- Miliauskas, G., Venskutonis, P. R., & Van Beek, T. A. (2004). Screening of radical scavenging activity of some medicinal and aromatic plant extracts. *Food chemistry, 85*(2), 231-237.

www.ingramcontent.com/pod-product-compliance
Lightning Source LLC
Chambersburg PA
CBHW070815250726
48662CB00004B/2054